WITHDRAWN

Cardiology

Two Week Loan

SELF-ASSESSMENT PICTURE TESTS IN MEDICINE

Cardiology

Dr Wajdi Turkie

Research Registrar
Manchester Heart Centre
The University of Manchester
The Royal Infirmary
Manchester, England

Dr Derek Rowlands

Consultant Cardiologist
Manchester Heart Centre
The University of Manchester
The Royal Infirmary
Manchester, England

Mosby-Wolfe

London Baltimore Barcelona Bogotá Boston Buenos Aires Caracas Carlsbad, CA Chicago Madrid Mexico City
Milan Naples, FL New York Philadelphia St. Louis Seoul Singapore Sydney Taipei Tokyo Toronto Wiesbaden

Project Managers:	Elaine Graham
	Paul Phillips
Editorial Assistant:	Sarah Edwards
Development Editor:	Jennifer Prast
Production:	Siobhan Egan
Index:	Angela Cottingham
Publisher:	Richard Furn

For full details of all Times Mirror International Publishers Limited titles, please write to Times Mirror International Publishers Limited, Lynton House, 7–12 Tavistock Square, London WC1H 9LB, England.

A CIP catalogue record for this book is available from the British Library.

Library of Congress Cataloging-in-Publication Data applied for.

PREFACE

Heart disease dominates the public's interest in health matters and inevitably intrudes into the experience of every practising doctor, whatever his or her discipline. The use of non-invasive investigations (especially electrocardiography, the chest x-ray and cardiac ultrasound) is now widespread and every new generation of doctors must learn these basic techniques.

The use of pictures is well recognised as a means of facilitating understanding and learning. We have provided here a collection of illustrations and comments, all highly pertinent to everyday cardiac problems. These should be helpful for medical students, newly qualified doctors and nurses, as well as for more experienced doctors whose primary clinical duties are not dominantly cardiac but for whom an understanding af basic cardiac investigations is essential (for example, general practitioners and general physicians). It is very much hoped that this publication will be helpful for many in those groups.

The authors would welcome comments and feedback which, if received, would certainly be taken into account in respect of any future publication.

Wajdi Turkie
Derek Rowlands

ACKNOWLEDGEMENTS

We gratefully acknowledge the contributions in terms of illustrations provided by our colleagues: Drs. W.C. Brownlee, A.P. Fitzpatrick, Professor P.N. Durrington, Mr. D. J. M. Keenan, Dr. J.C. Creamer and Dr. P. Bishop.

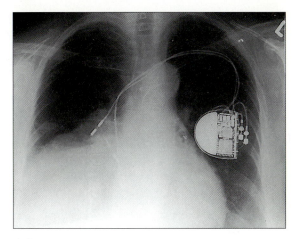

▲ 1

i. What type of heart transplant did this patient have?

ii. Why did the patient require a pacemaker?

iii. List four indications for this type of transplant procedure.

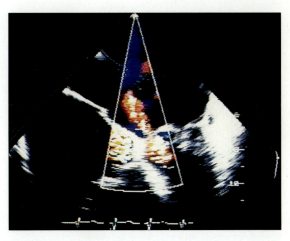

▲ 2

i. What abnormality is seen on this echocardiogram?

ii. What is the most likely cause?

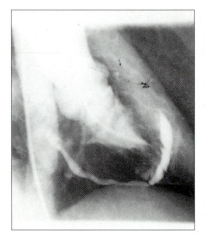

▲ 3
i. What procedure was carried out on this patient and what complication had occurred?
ii. How could you manage the patient?

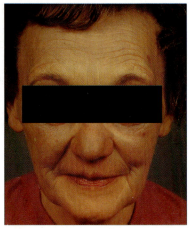

▲ 4
What abnormality is shown and what is the cause?

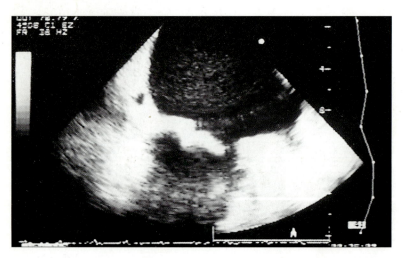

▲ 5
What abnormality is shown on this echocardiogram and what is the most likely cause?

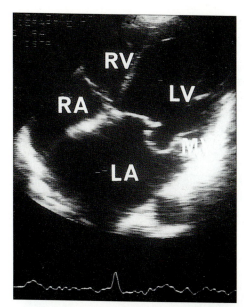

6

i. What abnormality is seen on this echocardiogram?

ii. Name four conditions associated with this abnormality.

iii. What is the arrhythmia most commonly associated with it?

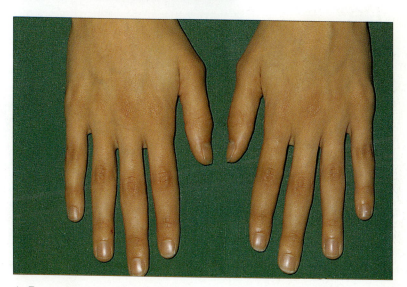

▲ **7**

What cardiological abnormalities are associated with this condition?

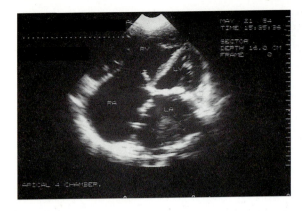

◀ 8
Describe the abnormalities seen on this transthoracic echocardiogram.

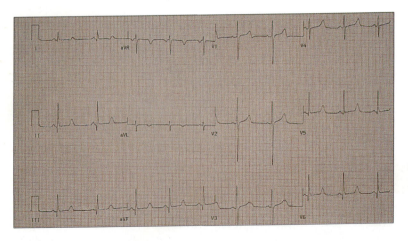

▲ 9
i.   What is the main abnormality on this ECG?
ii. List four conditions and four drugs that may cause this abnormality.

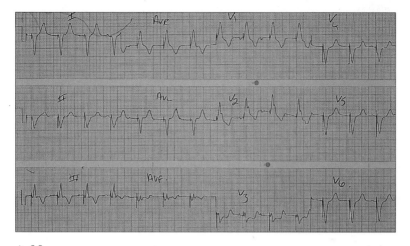

▲ 10

This ECG was taken two hours after a pacemaker was implanted. Describe
the abnormality and what caused it.

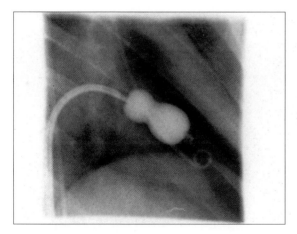

▲ 11

i. What procedure is the patient undergoing?
ii. List the complications that are associated with this
   procedure.

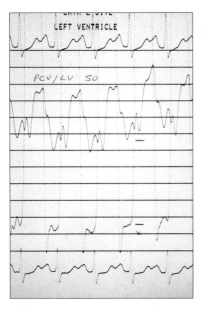

LEFT VENTRICLE

PCV/LV 50

◀ 12

These pressure tracings are from a patient complaining of marked breathlessness. The pressure scale is 5 mmHg per graduation.

i. What do the two pressures represent?
ii. What is the diagnosis?
iii. How would you treat the patient?

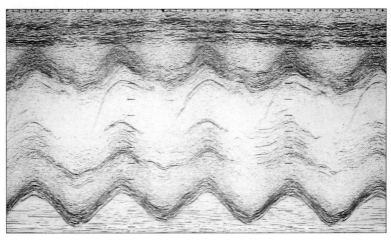

▲ 13

i. Identify the abnormality in this echocardiogram.
ii. List four common causes of this abnormality.